Vegan Aging 101

A Guide to Help you Look Younger, Have More Energy, and Live a Longer and Healthy Life the Vegan Way

Project Vegan

Table of Contents

Intro 1

Chapter 1: Diet, Aging, And "Inevitability" 3

Chapter 2: Pros And Cons Of Going Vegan 8

Chapter 3: The Animal Protein Myth 14

Chapter 4: How Do Your Dietary Needs Change
With Age? 18

Chapter 5: Drink More Water To Delay The Aging
Process 20

Chapter 6: Best Foods For Anti-Aging............................25

Chapter 7: Do Older Adults Have Special Nutritional
Needs? 30

Chapter 8: The Surprising Anti-Aging Benefits Of Fiber..32

Chapter 9: The Importance Of Whole Foods And Color
Variety 36

Chapter 10: Vegan Food Substitution Guide 40

Conclusion...43

Intro

Does the thought of aging worry you? If so, you are not alone. From old folktales about the fountain of youth to current promises of "miracle" anti-aging medicine. The truth is that people have sought to retain their youth since people first noticed they were aging. However, there is no miracle promise to aging. Those searching in vain for cures or shortcuts that make too good to be true promises are, unfortunately, missing the mark. Instead of trying to fight the process of aging through artificial measures, we should analyze what we eat on a daily basis. There are various anti-aging benefits to a vegan diet that can help you both feel and look younger. The goal should not be miracle cures but rather healthy living. As we age, we become less adept at proper hydration. A healthy adult's body contains around 60% water weight while an older adult is usually more like 55%. The effects of this decline in hydration are clear: drier, rougher skin and wrinkles, which is why often our skin glows less as we age. A key to avoiding such a descent, therefore, is do our best to stay hydrated.

A vegan diet is a fantastic way to avoid the aging induced by dehydration. Our bodies require a substantial amount of water, and vegan food choices are fairly water-rich. For example, vegan diets encourage you to grub on fresh fruits rather than processed, dry potato chips. Since the majority of the water we drink comes from what we eat, these changes add up to a lot more hydration and healthier, vibrant looking skin.

Another key contributor to our body's aging progression is a lack of various key vitamins, induced in large part by unhealthy eating habits. Vitamin C is one of those nutrients. Vitamin C destroys the unhealthy free radicals in your body. This damage is one of the main causes of aging. Vitamin C also destroys the free radicals and prohibits them from hurting you. Another Vitamin, Vitamin E, works as a fighting agent in our body's war against free radicals, encircling them so Vitamin C can destroy them.

People who practice a vegan diet benefit from eating many nutritious, age-defying foods of which many people on standard diets are deprived of. Your body will welcome this choice by preserving your youth longer and functioning better. And that is only one of the many benefits of veganism. Get ready to also have more energy and the ability to be more active throughout the day as well as contributing to a greener environment and living the most ethical lifestyle you possibly can.

Chapter 1
Diet, Aging, and "Inevitability"

There is no diet that will keep you young forever. It's an enticing promise and will certainly sell a good deal of books and diet plans, but it's simply a lie: Humans are very vulnerable to aging, and there are little to no ways to prevent that. No diet guarantees immortality. But appropriate nutrition can do wonders to avoid what can be avoided, instead of simply accepting it as a certain conclusion.

However, that doesn't mean you need to speed up your aging process. Accepting your limitations as a human is one thing, accepting premature ailment is completely different. Many people today simply accept all their health issues after 50 as "aging" and don't even consider attempting to change their dietary habits to handle those cramped knees, dodgy back, or bolstered beer belly.

Actually, the truth is these problems are linked to one's diet and are "inevitable" on a standard American diet that might not seem so inevitable to a person who practices a healthy diet. So, without trying to sell eternal youth, here is a quick breakdown of a few common signs and symptoms of aging that we consider unavoidable and how diet can help to minimalize them.

Bone aging

The major effect aging has on our body's bones is the loss of calcium homeostasis, which is critical to maintaining bone structure. As one ages, homeostasis is agitated, which results in the bones becoming more delicate. While the definite causes of the agitation are not clear, it has been noticed that bone detrition is more drastic in women than in men. In women, bones start losing calcium at around the age of 30. By age 70, women could lose up to 30% of their bone calcium. The majority of men don't start losing calcium until they reach the age of 60.

Moreover, the loss of calcium due to aging slows down protein synthesis. As a consequence, there is not much generation of collagen fibers. These fibers are needed to maintain the bones' strength and dexterity, and without them, bones turn frail, culminating in a higher chance of fracture.

Finally, bone retention occurspursues without the consequent formation of new bone tissue. As aa consequence, larger, centrally placed medullary cavities of compact bone the thinner walls of the compact bone become weaker.

Brain Aging

Do people inevitably become more absent-minded as they age? Maybe, but a lot of research also shows that it is dictated by diet. For example, a review by the Journal of Neuroscience shows the role of antioxidants from fruits, veggies and spices in averting age-related switches in the brain. Older adults usually have limited access to organic fruits and vegetables and seldom eat enough of them which raises the question: is mental detriment inevitable, or is it partially an outcome of diet?

Other likely important nutrients consist of Omega-3 fats and B vitamins. Supplements, in particular, have not culminated as researchers prospected. However, there is possibly some kind of synergy among the nutrients in whole foods that have yet to be replicated in any supplement form. Whatever the case, the research shows that a healthy and balanced diet is much better than white bread and a bunch of pills.

There's also a link in micronutrients. A standard American diet is very high in refined carbs and low in healthy fats and protein. This isn't necessarily a recipe for great metabolic health: it causes insulin resistance as well as other complications of carbohydrate metabolism. And those complications are a very important part of brain health, including major neurodegenerative diseases. Alzheimer's, in particular, is similar to Type 3 Diabetes – that is to say, an issue of carbohydrate metabolism.

This doesn't infer that "carbs are the cause of Alzheimer's," and it doesn't mean that improving metabolic health will impede or cure it, as neurological diseases are complex and are made up of various factors. But it does propose that the type of brain deterioration commonly found in a high-refined carb American diet might not be very preventable in people who practice a healthier diet.

Skin aging

Skin aging is the result of both natural aging and overexposure to sunlight. A hint of sunshine can do wonders, including helping to increase Vitamin D levels which helps fight depression among other things. However, absorbing too much has negative consequences for our skin.

Add this to the inevitable constant of aging, and the result is wrinkly and saggy skin: the signs of skin aging.

The skin has two different layers. The epidermis is the outer shield of our skin and guards us against environmental hazards, such as ultraviolet radiation and bacteria. Meanwhile, the dermis is loaded with collagens, which are the decisive factors in keeping our skin strong and elastic.

Both layers undergo a lot of stress during our lives, and as time goes by, permanent damage accumulates. But, is this damage permanent and unrepairable?

Dermal cells lose connections

The dermis contains a complex conglomerate of extracellular matrix (ECM) proteins, which include elastin and collagen, which keep your skin elastic.

Fibroblast cells not only generate these proteins, but they are also embedded in between these proteins and linked to them. As we get older, the ECM gradually deteriorates as the protein compounds become fragmented.

Fibroblasts lose ECMs as enzymes gradually deplete the protein networks. This results in a transformation of fibroblast shape, drastically damaging the cells' function. Protein creation by fibroblasts is decreased, further contributing to the disintegration of the ECM network.

This dramatic cycle of events causes a drastic reduction in elasticity and makes us lose our pert skin tone. Why this occurs during our aging process is not obvious, but researchers believe that it is a result of a combination of chronic inflammation and oxidative stress damage to DNA, cell senescence.

Fat tissue and aging

As our body ages, the fat below the skin manually shrinks, resulting in wrinkling and sagging. But as of recently, scientists could not find any correlation between UV damage and fat; UV rays do not infiltrate deep enough to contact the subcutaneous fat.

However, according to the NCBI, a newly discovered fat depot in the deep dermis was found to be able to infiltrate the upper dermis, which is well in the range of UV light.

These particular fat cells also reply to chemicals dispersed by cells in the epidermis. As a counter to severe UV damage, these fat cells die out, and scar tissue appears in their place.

Armed with this information, is it possible we can avoid the unavoidable accumulation of skin damage? Light sun exposure will certainly reduce the severity of damage that UV can inflict on your skin.

If you are eating vegan, you have likely got most of these checked, just refrain from too many nuts and seeds and vegan candy, and savor your good skin.

Chapter 2
Pros and Cons of Going Vegan

Possible benefits

A Vegan diet is generally healthier. Well-planned vegan diets are rich in protein, iron, calcium and other essential vitamins and minerals. These nutrients tend to be low in saturated fat, high in fiber and packed with antioxidants, which can negate some of the western world's biggest health related problems, like obesity, heart disease, diabetes and cancer. But that is not to say it is perfect without any drawbacks. Lets look into some of the benefits as well as cons.

Better Digestion

This is probably the most obvious one. Your digestion will SKY ROCKET on a vegan diet, no doubt. A vegan diet is rich in fiber, healthy fats, water and healthy plant-based protein. It has nothing that will get in the way of your digestion (unless maybe you opt for highly processed foods, which are harder for your stomach to break down). Just take some caution on fiber intake. Eating slowly and chewing your food well also helps with your digestion, in addition to curbing down hunger. Someone who comes from a habit of eating cheese, meat and milk will certainly benefit from a change to a vegan diet, as they will quickly see how it can heal chronic constipation, as well as keep you from feeling bloated or gassy, heal stomach inflammation, and cure even heart problems.

Obesity

Be it a young or an old individual, a vegan diet helps fight and avoid obesity. Many studies have shown that vegans, in comparison to people of different diet groups, are less prone to obesity and have lowest body mass index overall. The reason being is that a vegan's diet consists of much higher fiber foods and bad fats, such as saturated and trans fats. Instead, vegans turn to the healthier kind of Omega fats discussed earlier, which are found in nuts and natural oils, though they can lead to weight gain when taken excessively.

Skin

It's no secret, fruits and vegetables are your skin's best friends, so naturally a diet that revolves around them will do wonders for your skins health. Fat found in animal products causes excess oil production that can lead to clogged pores, which cause acne breakouts. Phytochemicals, enzymes, essential vitamins and antioxidants found in fruits and vegetables also help promote more radiant skin. While fiber found in whole grains also amplifies radiant skin by flushing out toxins. If you want maximum benefits to your skin, you might want to consider drastically upping your intake of raw fruits and veggies.

Better Sleep

Yes, sleep. Even though a vegan diet may keep you feeling energetic and rejuvenated all day, due to the slowly absorbed sugars in many whole foods, it also fights stress which allows you to sleep better. Plus, you can find a good supply of Vitamin B6, tryptophan, and magnesium in plant based foods that help you keep a healthy sleep cycle. These foods include: Sweet potatoes, cashew butter, peanut butter, bananas, broccoli, avocados, kale, almonds, squash, walnuts, and spinach. Meanwhile, calcium, which aids sleep, can also be found in foods such as almond or soy milk, Kale, Swiss chard, and dried figs, all of which are richer in calcium than dairy.

Less Inflammation

Inflammation is the body's immunity response to an apparent threat, but what is it that your body thinks is a threat? Initially, scientists thought that the inflammation from consuming meat may have been attributed to just animal protein. However, they also found that dairy products that are high in saturated fat also trigger an inflammatory response from the body. Further research showed that consuming a meal containing animal products causes bacterial toxins known as endotoxins to enter the bloodstream, that in turn trigger inflammation.

Plant based foods can help manage and lower inflammation. Inflammation is lowered particularly by food high in omega-3 fats like flax and Chia, coupled with chlorophyll found in leafy green vegetables. Legumes and dark green vegetables also increase body's alkalinity to calm down inflammation.

Possible Cons

Some people do find a vegan diet quite depriving, because they do not substitute their favorite foods correctly, or they do not look at it from a ethical perspective. But whether you are vegan for political, ethical or just health benefits, these are the common disadvantages with a vegan diet, as far as health is concerned.

Possibility of Lower Testosterone Levels

An increase in testosterone levels helps with muscle mass, energy levels, libido, strength, and body fat. Testosterone levels are mainly influenced by saturated fat and cholesterol in your diet. However, these are mainly available in meat and animal products. Aside from this, the amount of fiber in Vegan diets also reduces cholesterol and has been found to be linked to low testosterone levels.

However, in a study published by the British Journal of Cancer and The Oxford Vegetarian Study published by the American Journal of Nutrition, showed that a diet which also includes phytochemicals from fresh fruits and vegetables help increase testosterone. In these studies, vegetarians were found to have equal if not even higher testosterone levels than meat-eaters, with a plus of being at less risk of heart attack and prostate cancer.

Health Issues

Soy comes into the vegan diet quite often. It is high in the female hormone phytoestrogen. Eating small quantities is okay, just like they do in Asia, also you may want to reduce your intake even more for processed soy. As excess intake can cause cancer, infertility, heart disease, and gains in fat.

Potential shortage of certain vitamins

For the most part, plant based foods do not naturally contain B12, an essential nutrient. The only way is usually

B12 supplement or less healthier processed foods (such as soy milk, mock meats, cereals and brag's nutritional yeast) A vegan diet may also lack in vitamin D although there are vegan sources of these nutrients such as mushrooms and Vitamin D3 supplements.

Allergies

Having allergies to soy can prove to be quite a challenge on a vegan diet. It will be have to be cautious when consuming your products. Absolutely do not buy any packaged products without a nutrition label, and always be on the lookout for any of the following ingredients if you are allergic to soy:

- Edamame
- Kinako
- Nimame
- Okara
- Soya Natto
- Bean curd
- Yuba
- Soybean

Also lookout for the following as they may also have hidden sources of soy:

- Frozen desserts
- Seasoning & Spices
- Breaded foods

- Soups
- Beverage mixes
- MSG
- Chewing Gum
- Infant formula
- Cosmetics and soaps
- Dressings, gravies & marinades
- Baked goods

Chapter 3
The Animal Protein Myth

How much protein is enough to support muscle growth, or even just to have a long and healthy life? Here we will discuss the common misconceptions about plant proteins and complete versus incomplete proteins.

Very often, people have the idea that plant-based proteins are 'incomplete', making them poorer sources of protein than animal-based proteins. You will also notice that for plant-based proteins to be healthy and 'complete' they have to be taken in combinations which can make it a sophisticated approach.

However, what makes a protein actually "complete"? Proteins have the fundamental muscle building blocks known as amino acids. These components connect to conform proteins, similar to cars being connected to build a high speed train or maybe letters of the alphabet put together to create words.

The body has 21 various amino acids, nine of which are labeled essential; these are the ones the body cannot produce out of other amino acids, and so you need to supply them through the food that you consume on a daily basis. A 'complete' protein is one that has 9 fundamental amino acids (Leucine, Isoleucine, Lysine, Methionine, Phyenulanine, Thereonine, Tryptophan, Valine, and Histidine) required for the human body. In this sense, all plant-based protein you consume are a 'complete' protein.

However there is a possibility you might experience other imbalances in nutrients, to avoid this, just make sure you are consuming a wide variety of foods and make your plate as colorful as possible, and you have nothing to worry about!

Vegan Protein Sources

Here is a rundown of some of the more noticeable sources of vegan protein:

Green Peas

All foods in the legume family are great sources of vegan protein, and peas are no exception: 1 cup contains 7.9 grams—for comparison that is the same as 1 cup of dairy milk.

Quinoa

This grain is so healthy and delicious that NASA is trying to harvest it for current space missions. Packed with fiber, magnesium, iron, manganese, and of course protein, this grain a great replacement for rice and it's versatile enough to be used as main dish, such as casseroles, or sweet snacks like muffins, fritters and cookies.

Hempseed

This superfood seed has all 9 required amino acids, in addition to plenty of zinc, magnesium, iron, protein, and calcium. As a bonus, these seeds are also a source of essential fatty acids like omega-3's, which are great for overall health and lowering inflammation, as noted earlier.

Soy

Sure this protein has a negative connotation due to it increasing levels of estrogen and possibly being unhealthy when in processed form. However soy is a complete protein and rightfully deserves its status as the main substitute for meat-free products. Tofu is probably the best known soy product. Since we are concerned about protein mainly, it's ideal to choose the firmest tofu possible—the harder the, the higher the protein content.

Lentils

Lentils are essential and can easily be prepared to be eaten on a regular basis. They have a generous amount of protein, as well as being one of the highest alkalizing foods on the planet.

Lentils are also packed with a ton of fiber, in a single 100 gram serving you get 26 grams of protein as well as also meeting your entire daily value of fiber. Due to this, lentils are very satiating, so you probably will not be able to eat a huge serving size in a single sitting, but adding just a small amount of lentils to your diet is very beneficial.

Black beans

Beans are an essential in most vegan diets, being a part of popular dishes like burritos and black bean burgers, vegans have known what a great source of protein they are for quite some time.

One of the particular health benefits of black beans is their ability to fight diabetes, as they help maintain healthy blood sugar levels. They also help the digestive tract because of their high ratio of protein and fiber, and their lack of fats.

Nuts and Nut Butters

A small batch of cashews, walnuts or almonds provide a quick-and-easy protein fix. Nut butter is great for making your own homemade protein bars (Check the bonus protein bar chapter in this book) or a quick spreaded toast. Indeed nuts are a great on the go way of getting a rich nutritional fix.

Greens

Lastly, greens provide a flavorful and nutritious dose of protein to compliment any dish. It's never a bad time to get some extra greens into your diet. A single cup of Spinach has 7 whole grams of protein, and it's dark leafy green relative kale packs 3 grams per each cup. I f you would like to mask the taste, there are tons of ways you can mix greens into a shake, they go great with bananas, soymilk and even apples. Even just cooking a handful of delicious kale chips can give you a fix of delicious protein.

Chapter 4
How Do Your Dietary Needs Change with Age?

As you get older in age, your eating habits, nutritional needs and appetite can shift in many ways. Some people notice their appetite starts dropping as they age. Lowering your calorie intake can make it more problematic to get the necessary nutrients to maintain muscle and bone health.

Staying physically active will help boost your appetite. But if perhaps you are not a heavy eater and would rather take it easy, you should still stick to a healthy and balanced diet.

That's because aging is related to various changes, which include decreased quality of life, nutrient deficiencies and poor health outcomes. Fortunately, there are ways you can help prevent age-related changes. For example, eating nutritious foods and exercising regularly can help you stay healthy as you age.

This chapter will explain your nutritional needs and how they change as you age, as well as how to address them.

Appetites

Many people start losing their appetite as they age. It is also natural for your sense of smell and taste to diminish which can result in you eating less.

If you're burning fewer calories through exercise or physical activity, it may be a good idea to eat less. However, you still need to consume enough nutrients and minerals to maintain healthy bones, organs and muscle. Not eating enough can result in health problems and malnutrition.

Medical Conditions

As you age, you become more vulnerable to health problems, like diabetes, high cholesterol, high blood pressure and osteoporosis. To reduce the chance of these conditions, your physician may recommend switching up your diet.

For example, if you have diabetes, high cholesterol or high blood pressure, you can eat foods that are low in calories but rich in nutrients. Your physician may also suggest that you consume less sodium.

Many older adults develop a sensitivity to foods such as peppers, onions and spicy foods. You may need to eliminate these foods from your diet.

Calories

You will require fewer calories as you age to retain a healthy weight. Consuming lots of calories without adequate exercises leads to weight gain. You may also become energy deficient and experience more muscle problems as you get older. As a result, it will be harder for you to burn off calories through exercise or physical activity. You may also experience loss in muscle mass, which results in your metabolism slowing down, decreasing your caloric needs.

Chapter 5
Drink More Water to Delay the Aging Process

As you grow older, you don't drink as much water because you don't often feel as thirsty as you used to in your early twenties.

If you do not drink a sufficient amount of water, you will experience dehydration which is echoed in your skin, it also affects your digestive track, and you become constipated as well as tired and fatigued. The combined outcome of all this makes you feel and look older than you really should. This is how important the role of water is to our overall health and aging development.

Stay Hydrated

When the temperature is high, getting properly hydrated is crucial, regardless of whether you are physically active or just laying on a sunny beach.

Not drinking a large glass of water before a morning run, sweating excessively during workouts, and withstanding hot temperatures are sure ways to become dehydrated. Consuming water during exercising can also aid in battling fatigue and extend your endurance.

How to Determine if You Are Hydrated

Below are some ways to determine if you are appropriately hydrated.

Urine color

Your urine color can be a good sign. If it is a clean water color, then the likelihood that you are hydrated is very high. If the color is dark or has a strange odor, that is an indicator that you are dehydrated. Please note that consuming a B12 supplement can have an impact on your urine color, but this does not mean you are dehydrated. However, always check with your doctor if you are suspicious about anything.

Rate of Sweat

Another method to determine your hydration level is to check your weight before and after working out. The before/after hydrating weight difference will provide you with a sign of your hydration level. If you have added or kept the same weight, you could conclude that you're hydrated. If you are down in weight by a noticeable amount, you will need to drink more water to restore the weight you have lost.

What's the amount of water you should be drinking?

The amount of water you should take differs; a person who sweats significantly should drink higher amounts than someone who doesn't. This is especially true for athletes who train during the hot summer months. For every pound of sweat lost, that's a pint of water you will need to recuperate. This is why it's not strange for a high school football player with pads and running drills to drop five pounds of sweat while practicing during the summer.

Create a hydration habit

Some people work so hard to the point where they hardly have any time to eat, or even catch a regular water break. But making a habit of being hydrated will aid you in maintaining your energy and attention so that your body and mind can function optimally. Below are some tips for getting your fluid fix throughout the day much easier

Always have water on hand, even if you are at work

If you keep a bottle of water near you, it will make it more convenient to sip water throughout the day, without it seeming like a drag. If you start to feel nauseous or fatigued, drink some cold water. It's a quick way to make you more alert anytime you are in a slump.

Eat lots of whole foods

Wholefoods naturally contain water and will drastically increase your fluid levels, as opposed to processed foods which contain little to no water and will leave you dehydrated and fatigued.

Mix it up

Does H20 seem boring? Here are some tips on how you can get other sources of water.

Fuse it

Cut fruit slices, such as lime, oranges and lemon in a water container and let refrigerate for a few hours.

Add coconut ice cubes

Add the coconut water to your ice cube tray, then scoop the ice cubes in a glass of water for a sweet and nutty taste.

Sip herbal tea

Try sipping on a cup of herbal tea every day. If you do this regularly, you'll have the additional fluids of 1 cup of water to your tally every day. In addition, this can be a therapeutic way to let go of stress at the day's end.

Eat rice

Rice has super absorbent components which work as a strong tool to replenish you with fluids after it has been cooked in water. It also has the added benefit of boosting your energy through carbs. However, stay away from overtly salty rice dishes, as excess sodium retains water and will make you feel bloated and sluggish.

Eat your water

Try eating these foods for a delicious and simple way of increasing your H20 absorption without directly drinking water.

1 medium apple = 6 ounces

1 cup of watermelon balls

1 navel orange = 4 ounces

1 cup uncooked broccoli florets = 2 ounces

1 cup cooked chopped3zuccini = 6 ounces

1 cup chopped cantaloupe = 5 ounces

10 baby carrots = 3 ounces

Not sweating during hardcore exercise can be a sign that you are hydrated to the point of exhaustion due to the heat. Also, you should be careful of sugary drinks or fruit juices and soda, as they can be harsh on your stomach if you are not hydrated. It's also advisable to stay away from drinks that are made up of caffeine, which can perform as a diuretic and result in the loss of more fluids.

Now that you understand the impact that hydration can have on you, remember that you will not have to worry if you drink at least 11 cups a day as part of your daily habit.

Chapter 6
Best Foods for Anti-aging

Your middle age and beyond. Anti-aging researchers agree that eating plenty of mono-saturated fats, antioxidants and omega-3 fats can help you to maintain good health and look great and youthful throughout the years. Eat the following foods which are all rich in most essential nutrients. They're easily incorporated into your diet and taste good to boot!

Berries

Berries are loaded with polyphenols that are known to protect against age-related switches in the brain. Polyphenols function in two ways. First, they delegate an electron to free harmful radicals in the brain, which negates the radicals and sways them from undermining the brain cell membranes. Also, polyphenols negate the body's compound production which causes inflammation and, in turn, enables the formation of amyloid plaques that harm the brain by eliminating neurons. Cranberries, cherries and prunes are also comprised of these protective polyphenol antioxidants.

Garlic

Garlic contains a nutrient called allicin that protects the heart in various important ways. Garlic helps to decrease blood cholesterol levels, delays the hardening of the arteries and creation of atherosclerosis by reducing blood thickness. Research has also shown that garlic is a contributing factor in lowering blood pressure. Lower blood pressure and thinner blood permit the blood flow to move more freely through our arteries, making tiny tears and other artery damages much less likely to occur and decreasing the probability of low blood flow to the heart.

Turmeric

Turmeric, an essential in Indian cuisine, may be beneficial to our immune system. Studies show that turmeric may counter the development of autoimmune diseases such as rheumatoid arthritis. When the immune system is overworked, it often turns on itself, attacking and destroying its own tissues, which is what happens with arthritis. Studies also show that curcumin may boost the immune system. This not only helps to prevent osteoarthritis, but also helps fend off infection—especially as we get older and our immune system becomes less efficient.

Beans

Beans are an anti-aging super force because they are packed with lignans, a kind of phytoestrogen that helps to prevent breast cancer in women past menopause. In one new study done by BreastCancer.org, women who followed a diet rich in lignans had a 17 percent decline in breast cancer risk. Lignans help shelter the body from toxins, xenoestrogens, plastics and other environmental components that imitate natural estrogens. These inflict damage on the endocrine system and increase the probability of hormonal cancers. Lignans also help to defend against various other cancers like colon cancer.

Tomatoes

Tomatoes are loaded in lycopene, a fairly rare antioxidant that prevents cardiovascular disease by dropping cholesterol. A recent study by the NCBI concluded that eating tomato paste drastically lowers high LDL levels and boosts good LDL levels. Tomato lycopene also minimizes the risk of stroke and heart attack by preventing clotting in similar ways that aspirin does—without any of the adverse side effects. Other studies concluded that tomatoes minimalize the probability of breast and prostate cancer, and prevent skin damage from sun exposure. Studies have shown that tomato paste cooked with olive oil is the most beneficial because cooking and processing it dissolves the tomatoes cells and makes the lycopene more accessible.

Spinach

Spinach contains carotenoids, a plant component that has powerful antioxidant value. One of these carotenoids, lutein, is most notably helpful in defending our eyes from macular degeneration. Researchers believe it works by delegating an electron to non-harmful radicals in the eyes lens, which reduces the risk of damage. In an identical way, carotenoids also eliminate free radicals in the skin, which stagnates the aging process—and the visibility of wrinkles. Other leafy, dark green vegetables such as chard, collards and kale are also rich in carotenoids, as are red-orange fruits and veggies like carrots, red bell peppers, and pumpkin.

Green tea

Green tea contains epigallocatechin gallate (ECGC), another strong polyphenol antioxidant that prevents the growth and formation of tumors and boosts death in cancer cells. As time goes by, free radical deterioration can damage our body's cells and make them lose their capacity to balance division and growth; the result is cancer. ECGC functions by connecting to free radicals, which prevent them from destroying the cells' DNA. A recent study discovered that green tea also guards against sun-related skin cancers by decreasing the DNA destruction inflicted by UVB rays. Another impressive discovery is the power of EGCG to rejuvenate dying skin cells, a discovery that might benefit skin illnesses like psoriasis, rosacea, wounds, ulcers—and yes, also wrinkles. Green tea is optimal when caffeinated, as the decaffeination procedure abolishes about 50 percent of the guarding antioxidants together with caffeine, which research has shown may also guard against sun-related skin cancers and damage.

Dark Leafy Greens

Research shows that Vitamin E may serve as a key protector from pro-inflammatory molecules known as inflammatory cytokines which negatively affect the body. One of the ideal sources of Vitamin E are dark green vegetables, such as kale, spinach, collard greens and broccoli. Dark greens also usually contain a higher consolidation of vitamins and minerals—like iron, calcium and disease deterring phytochemicals—than their lighter colored leaf counterparts.

Cruciferous vegetables

Cruciferous vegetables, such as kale and broccoli, contain a chemical mineral called diindolylmethane (DIM), which research shows shields women against aging hormonal changes. As the body ages, its ability to dissolve estrogen tends to decrease. DIM helps the body dissolve estrogen into a more secure, usable form, so it transforms into a protective compound against breast and reproductive organ cancers. Cruciferous veggies are also loaded in indole-3-carbinol, a powerful cancer-preventive nutrient. Studies show that it hinders the growth and multiplication of cancer cells and helps maintain pre-cancerous cells from further developing.

Chapter 7
Do Older Adults Have Special Nutritional Needs?

Not much information is available with regard to how aging impacts an individual's body's ability to absorb and hold onto vitamins and minerals. Therefore, we do not have much knowledge regarding how the nutritional requirements of younger adults change from those of older adults. The ideal nutrient intake for older adults is directly derived from the exact intake of younger adults.

One approach that is generally agreed upon, however, is that older people usually take in fewer calories and energy then they require. This may be due, in part, by a decrease in people's metabolism as they age. It might also reflect a drop in physical activity if the total consumption of carbs, protein, fat and vitamins also decline. If calorie intake is not enough, then consumption of excess nutrients might also be required.

Various other aspects can adjust the nutritional requirements of older adults and how well they achieve those goals, such as what kind of food they have access to. For example, people aging can experience changes in the types of foods they are able to tolerate as well as changes in their ability to shop for or make food.

Generally, the dietary recommendations for young adults apply to older adults. Here is a summary of some of those foods:

Limit

- Sweets
- Greasy or fatty foods
- Alcohol
- Oil, and "junk" foods
- Added fat
- Regular coffee and tea
- Excessive salt

Eat plenty of

- Vegetables
- Fruits
- Whole grain breads and cereals

Drink

- Plenty of water and other fluids

Chapter 8
The Surprising Anti-Aging Benefits of Fiber

Fiber has a well-earned reputation for maintaining the digestive system in good functioning order – but it also does a lot more. In fact, it is one of the main players in many of your body's structures that help keep you youthful. For example, older adults who ate high fiber diets have an 80% higher chance of living longer and staying healthier than people who didn't, according to research done by the Journals of Gerontology.

The problem is that very few Americans eat the amount of fiber they should. For adults, 51 and older, US government guidelines suggest at least 28g daily for men and 22g for women.

What is Fiber Anyway?

Fiber is a carb found in plant foods: fruit, beans, nuts, grains and vegetables. Technically, carbs are not a nutrient because they are not broken down and dissolved, but that is why they are so beneficial to our health.

There are various types of fiber, and they all fit into two groups: soluble and insoluble.

Soluble fiber is delicate and fluidifies in water, creating a gel-like substance. It firms your stool, which results in an easier passage. Sources include legumes, beans, sweet potatoes, oats, and various fruits.

How fiber keeps you young

The study referenced previously followed 1,600 physically fit adults for 10 years. Those who aged without any major health problems (meaning they were free of cancer, diabetes, and heart disease), as well as maintaining good overall cardiovascular, physical and cognitive function at an average of 29g of fiber daily. How is it possible that this single substance can have such an impactful effect on health and endurance? It so happens that there are various ways fiber acts as an anti-aging miracle.

Cutting cholesterol: Soluble fiber connects to bile acids, liver produced fluids that aid in fat absorption and digestion, and it helps your body to expel them. After that, the body demands more bile acids, and it takes cholesterol from the blood to make some. A 2016 Cochrane Review of 23 tests discovered that boosting fiber led to a 7.7 mg/dl cutback in cholesterol and a 5.4 mg/dl decline in bad cholesterol.

Protecting against diabetes

A study done in 2009 by Diabetes Care discovered that people who ate less than 20g of fiber daily were about 50 percent more likely of contracting Type 2 diabetes than those who ate 61g or more daily. It also showed that eating high fiber foods delays the absorption of carbs into your bloodstream, so as a result, blood sugar levels spike at a slower rate and the pancreas is allowed more time to respond and produce insulin

Controlling weight

Fiber bulks up quickly, so you are satiated much faster and remain so longer. And many fiber-rich foods are also calorically diluted.

Lowering colon cancer risk

A recent study done by the American Institute for Cancer Research and the World Cancer Research Fund International concluded that eating 90g of high fiber whole grains per day could reduce colon cancer risk by 17 percent.

Reducing inflammation

Chronic inflammation has been associated with various diseases such as Alzheimer's, certain cancers, and even arthritis. Many studies have concluded that elevated insoluble fiber consumption leads to lower inflammation. This may be because of the other favorable nutrients of whole grains, such as magnesium and polyphenols.

Protecting joints

If fiber reduces inflammation, there is a possibility that it helps lower the risk of arthritis. And a study done by the Annals of the Rheumatic Diseases confirms this theory. Researchers looked over two groups of people and discovered that in one group, individuals who ate a daily fiber amount of around 20g had a 30 percent lower probability of osteoarthritis in the knee than those who consumed around 8g. While in the other group, those who consumed an average of 25g of fiber daily had a 61 percent lower probability in comparison with those who ate about 14g.

Boosting good bacteria in the gut

Fiber ferments when it reaches the colon. Instead of digesting, the fermented compound supplies food to aid the good bacteria to duplicate and thrive. A healthy amount of healthy bacteria can have long-reaching health effects, such as helping to control inflammation and strengthening the immune system.

Make sure to increase your fiber consumption gradually, and distribute it generously across meals, and also make sure to drink a lot of water, as without sufficient water, fiber can actually trigger constipation. It's also worth trying a variety of fiber-rich foods and settling on the ones which your digestive system processes the best.

Chapter 9
The Importance of Whole Foods and Color Variety

So, to carry out a plant-based diet properly, consume foods that are the least deviated from their natural state as possible. A broad range of whole plant foods in as many colors as you can will ensure you are attaining lots of rich minerals, vitamins, antioxidants, amino acids, proteins, and phytonutrients. Consumption of colorful foods like vegetables, dark-colored fruits, green tea, and berries can aid in the reduction of the probability of disease, quick recovery and safeguard cellular health.

A great place to begin is consuming a broad range of vegetables. I always suggest consumption of one large raw salad daily. It can be loaded up with as many vegetables as you prefer, then a few healthy fats like avocado and hemp seed can be added. You can also add a little protein like edamame or lentils if required, which can then be topped using apple cider vinegar or fat-free dressing.

Use the five-ingredient rule

If there is an excess of five ingredients on a nutrition label, it is a clear sign of an overly processed food, so try to avoid these. This will be the easiest and most straightforward way of preventing impulse buying on most unhealthy processed foods.

Stick to whole grains

Whole grain pasta, whole grain bread and whole grain cereal, you get the idea. No need to get rid of the carbs, in fact, you should embrace them as they are fundamental to a healthy vegan diet. Eating clean just means understanding which carbs are best for you. Whole grain is always a safe bet.

Revamp your food environment

It might be time to clear out your cupboards. One great way to ensure you don't consume junk food is to keep it out of your home altogether. Like most addictions, the best way to get it out of your life is to nip it in the bud.

You can't eat junk food if it is not there, and when it is an inconvenience to go to the store for a late-night snack, you will ask yourself if it is worth the effort. Once you create a healthy food environment, you will grow accustomed to loving the foods you are surrounded by.

Mistakes happen

Most changes are difficult and letting go of unhealthy addictive food is a tough change for most people. If you give in occasionally and eat junk foods, don't blame yourself and give up. After all, we are human, and this is a transitional process; we can always turn a mistake into a learning opportunity. Remember, you do not need to be perfect to succeed, so strive to make whole foods the central part of your diet slowly but surely.

Anti-inflammatory foods

Around 12.9 million people around the world have lost their lives due to some cardiovascular disease, according to statistics from the World Health Organization in 2012. It is estimated that each year, about eight million people lose their lives to cancer. Cancer and heart disease are expected to remain as the primary cause of death in developed countries following a western diet for many years to come.

To increase your odds of preventing these common health hazards, it's recommended to add anti-inflammatory foods to your diet. Below, we have a list of the recommended foods that are essential inflammatory preventers.

Fruits, veggies and starches

Again, we always want to go for diverse foods with lots of colors. Leafy greens are rich in vitamin K, and like kale and spinach, minimize inflammation, as do cabbage and broccoli. Meanwhile, whole grains like brown rice, whole-wheat bread, oatmeal and other grains that are unrefined have higher levels of fiber, which may also aid with inflammation.

Dark leafy greens

Studies have shown that Vitamin E plays a major role in protecting the body from inflammatory molecules known as cytokines, and one of the most beneficial sources of this vitamin are dark green veggies like kale, collard greens, and spinach. Dark greens also have the probability to have elevated concentrations of minerals and vitamins like iron, calcium, and disease-battling phytochemicals which their counterparts with lighter color lacks.

Tomatoes

Juicy red tomatoes are potent in lycopene which has been proven to minimize inflammation in the body and all through the lungs. Tomatoes that have been well cooked produce a higher level of lycopene than raw ones, so tomato sauce functions very well.

Ginger and turmeric

Turmeric functions in the body by assisting to put off NF-kappa B which is a protein that aids in regulating the immune system and triggers the inflammation process. Ginger, on the other hand, has been proven to minimize inflammation in the intestines when taken in the form of supplements.

Berries

Known as the superstars of the fruit and medicine world, berries are unique due to their elevated content of both antioxidants and fiber, like quercetin which is a flavonoid compound that provides support for a healthy growth of bacteria in the gut and averts damage to the colon. Berries have also been proven to slow mental decline and enhance memory function.

If you are allergic to any of the food stated here, it is best you avoid them regardless of how much nutrients they come with. Ingesting food that is sensitive to you will only result in more inflammation instead of reducing it.

Chapter 10
Vegan Food Substitution Guide

Being vegan does not mean you have to let go of your favorite homemade recipes and comfort foods. Fortunately, thanks to the rising popularity of veganism, many companies are creating vegan substitutes of their most popular food products. These are constantly evolving and improving in the modern age, which makes being vegan very convenient!

Cheese

When buying vegan cheese, check the label no matter what the cheese is labeled, as some contain casein which is an animal by-product. There are a wide variety of vegan cheeses such as Swiss, sliced and parmesan which you can use in the same way you would dairy cheese. If the faux-cheese taste is not to your liking for whatever reason, you may want to add some salt or herbs to spice up the taste.

Honey

While the ethical use of honey is debated in the vegan community, it cannot be argued that the bee population is decreasing. The best way to not contribute to this is obviously by not taking their food away. A bee makes honey to feed themselves primarily for survival. Fortunately, there are various replacements for honey such as maple syrup, agave nectar or date paste. All of these stand alone for their compatible sweetness to honey as well as their health benefits.

Milk

Perhaps the most simple food to substitute is milk. In fact, there are more vegan variations of milk than there are regular, which include: rice, soy, almond and oat milk. As for butternut milk, add 1 tbsp of vinegar in a measuring container and mix in soy or any non-dairy milk variety you desire or as the recipe specifies to make your own homemade variety.

Eggs

One of the best alternatives to scrambled eggs is tofu. You can choose to make it on your own through a recipe, or purchase tofu scrambler which you add with the tofu while cooking. You might make this a staple of your diet if you consume a diet high in protein.

Meat

Lastly but probably the most important staple of vegan foods are meat substitutes. Pretty much any meat based meal can easily be veganized. Sure it can be a bit inconvenient because you will be making a recipe from scratch, but the health and ethical benefits are worth it. Check out brands like Morningstar, Boca Burger and Toffuti for veganized versions of all your favorite foods!

As you can see, veganizing any dish is a snap once you are familiar with the substitutes. Plus cooking and preparing your own food can be quite therapeutic and fulfilling. Add to that the countless amazing health, ethical and environmental benefits and veganism will seem like anything but a drag!

Looking for veganized versions of animals products is probably the most difficult part of preparing vegan foods, especially if you are just trying these foods out for the first time. But it can also be exciting to mix up some long-held eating habits and getting amazing health benefits in the process. All it takes is a stroll down your local supermarket or health food aisle and you can see all the veganized substitutes for yourself.

Conclusion

There you have it. You are now well on your way to healthy aging the great Vegan way!

Be prepared to feel great, have energy you never had before and have the healthiest aging experience of your life! Thank you for taking the time to read my book and stay tuned for more books on Veganism in the future.

Thank you for reading! If you enjoyed my book and would recommend it to anyone. I'd be very grateful if you can leave a short review on Amazon. Your feedback is really important and I will use the opportunity to find out how I can improve this book even more.

Thanks again for your support!